ONKOLOGIE

Supplement 2, zu Band 24,
Februar 2001

Fatigue and Cancer
Fatigue und Krebs

Abstracts

2. Internationales Symposium
Köln, 16.–17. 2. 2001

Herausgeber

H. Flechtner
J.-U. Rüffer
Köln

Eine Veranstaltung der
Universitätskliniken zu Köln
Klinik I für Innere Medizin (Univ. Prof. V. Diehl)
Klinik für Kinder- und Jugendpsychiatrie (Univ. Prof. G. Lehmkuhl)
zusammen mit der
Arbeitsgemeinschaft Psychoonkologie (PSO)
der Deutschen Krebsgesellschaft (DKG)
und

ORTHO BIOTECH
Division of Janssen-Cilag GmbH,
Raiffeisenstrasse 8, 41470 Neuss, Germany

DEUTSCHE
KREBSGESELLSCHAFT E.V.

Universität
zu Köln

KARGER
Basel · Freiburg · Paris · London · New York ·
New Delhi · Bangkok · Singapore · Tokyo · Sydney

Bibliographische Dienste

Biological Abstracts
Current Contents/Clinical Medicine
Excerpta Medica/EMBASE
Index Medicus/MEDLINE
Medical Documentation Service
Reference Update
Research Alert
Science Citation Index
SCISEARCH Database

S. Karger · Medical and Scientific Publishers · Basel · Freiburg · Paris · London · New York · New Delhi · Bangkok · Singapore · Tokyo · Sydney

Die Zeitschrift erscheint zweimonatlich; pro Jahr erscheint 1 Band zu je 6 Heften. Mitglieder der Deutschen Gesellschaft für Hämatologie und Onkologie sowie der Österreichischen Gesellschaft für Hämatologie und Onkologie erhalten die Zeitschrift im Rahmen ihrer Mitgliedschaft. Der Bezug ist im Rahmen des Mitgliedbeitrags abgegolten. Bezugspreis für Jahrgang 24, 2001, DEM 238,– / CHF 179,–, einschließlich MwSt., zuzüglich Postgebühren. Der Abonnementpreis ist im voraus zahlbar. Das Abonnement der Zeitschrift läuft weiter, wenn es nicht spätestens 4 Wochen vor Abschluß eines Bandes abbestellt wird. Abonnementbestellungen können bei jeder Buchhandlung oder direkt beim Verlag aufgegeben werden:

Deutschland:
S. Karger GmbH
Lörracher Str. 16 a
D-79115 Freiburg
Tel. +49 7 61 45 20 70
Fax +49 7 61 4 52 07 14
E-mail Information@Karger.de

Übrige Länder:
S. Karger AG
Allschwilerstr. 10
Postfach
CH-4009 Basel
Tel. +41 61 3 06 11 11
Fax +41 61 3 06 12 34
E-mail Karger@Karger.ch

Anzeigen:
S. Karger
Verlag für Medizin und Naturwissenschaften GmbH,
Lörracher Str. 16 a, D-79115 Freiburg,
Tel. +49 7 61 45 20 70.
Gültig ist die Preisliste Nr. 11 vom 1. Januar 2001.

Supplement 2 zu Band 24, Februar 2001
ISBN 3-8055-7231-X

Verlagsleitung und presserechtlich verantwortlich:
Sibylle Hopf
Anzeigenleitung: Susanne Meister
Produktionsleitung: Georg Brunner

Satz und Druck: Walter Biering GmbH, Grafischer Betrieb
Freisinger Landstr. 21, D-80939 München

KARGER

Fax +49 761 4 52 07 14
E-mail Information@Karger.de
www.karger.com

Home Page der Zeitschrift:
www.karger.com/journals/onk

Band 24, Supplement 2, Februar 2001

Offizielles Organ der Deutschen Gesellschaft für Hämatologie und Onkologie,
der Österreichischen Gesellschaft für Hämatologie und Onkologie,
der Österreichischen Krebsgesellschaft – Krebsliga unter Fortführung der
«Österreichischen Zeitung für Onkologie»

ONKOLOGIE

• International Journal for Cancer Research and Treatment

KARGER

Basel · Freiburg · Paris · London · New York ·
New Delhi · Bangkok · Singapore · Tokyo · Sydney

ONKOLOGIE

Vol. 24, Suppl 2, Februar 2001

Wissenschaftliches Programm

Freitag, 16. 02. 2001

Workshop «Assessment and Intervention Strategies»

Methodik
Vorsitz: V. Diehl, R. Schwarz

Begrüßung
V. Diehl, Köln

Grußwort des Dekans der medizinischen Fakultät
G. Lehmkuhl, Köln

Einführung
J. Weis, Freiburg/Berlin

Das Konzept «Fatigue»
H. Flechtner, Köln

The measurement of fatigue over time: response shift in cancer patients
M. R M. Visser, Amsterdam (NL)

Ätiologie, Epidemiologie, Differentialdiagnose
Vorsitz: J. Weis, M. Heim

Fatigue und Zytokine
A. Josting, Köln

Das «Normwertproblem» – Fatigue in verschiedenen Bevölkerungsgruppen
R. Schwarz, Leipzig

Factors influencing fatigue after cure
M. Henry-Amar, Caen (F)

Fatigue und/oder Depression – Zur Differentialdiagnose von Fatigue
K. Reuter, Freiburg

The results of a systematic review of r-HuEPO on fatigue in cancer patients
A. Bottomley, Brüssel (B)

Tumoroxygenierung
Vorsitz: H. Flechtner, J.-U. Rüffer

Tumorhypoxie – Fakten, neue Erkenntnisse und der Einfluss der Anämie
P. Vaupel, Mainz

Tumoroxygenierung und Hämoglobin
A. Dietz, Heidelberg

Anämiekorrektur bei Patienten mit NSCLC unter multimodaler Therapie
W. Eberhardt, Essen

Der Hb-Wert als prognostischer Parameter für das Überleben von Tumorpatienten mit Kopf-/Hals-karzinomen
V. Budach, Berlin

Influence of Erythropoietin therapy on quality of life and survival of tumor patients under chemotherapy
T. J. Littlewood, Oxford (UK)

Keynote Lecture

Fatigue assessment in multi-lingual clinical trials
D. Cella, Evanston (USA)

KARGER

Fax +49 761 4 52 07 14
E-mail Information@Karger.de
www.karger.com

Artikel (Volltext) und Inhaltsverzeichnisse sowie das vorläufige Inhaltsverzeichnis des nächsten Heftes:
www.karger.com/journals/onk/onk_bk.htm

Vol. 24, Suppl 2, Februar 2001

Samstag, 17. 02. 2001

Klinik I
Vorsitz: M. Heim, J.-U. Rüffer

Fatigue and bone marrow transplantation – Current status and future directions
M. A. Andrykowski, Lexington (USA)

Fatigue in der Rehabilitation von Tumorpatienten
M. Heim, Bad Sooden

Prevalence and characteristics of fatigue in Hodgkin's disease survivors
J. H. Loge, Oslo (N)

Fatigue in long-term survivors
H. Knobel, Trondheim (N)

Hämoglobinwerte und subjektive Bewertung unter Chemotherapie
B. Holzner, Innsbruck (A)

Keynote Lecture

Clinical Issues
S. Kaasa, Trondheim (N) / Harvard (USA)

Klinik II
Vorsitz: R. Schwarz, H. Flechtner

Fatigue und Neuropsychologie
J. Weis, Freiburg/Berlin

Intervention bei Fatigue – ein mögliches Modell
J.-U. Rüffer, Köln

Behandlung von Fatigue bei Krebspatienten – Ausdauertraining als (Früh-)Rehabilitation
F. Dimeo, Berlin

Aerobic exercise training reduces fatigue in chronic fatigued Hodgkin´s disease survivors
L. M. Oldervoll, Trondheim (N)

Bericht vom Workshop «Assessment and Intervention Strategies»
H. Flechtner/J.-U. Rüffer, Köln

Zusammenfassung und Abschlussdiskussion
J. Weis, Freiburg/Berlin

ONKOLOGIE
Vol. 24, Suppl 2, Februar 2001

Referenten und Vorsitzende

Michael A. Andrykowski, PhD
Department of Behavioral Science
University of Kentucky
Lexington, KY, USA

Andrew Bottomley, PhD
Coordinator Quality of Life Unit
EORTC Data Center
Bruxelles, Belgium

Professor Dr. med. Volker Budach
Klinik für Strahlentherapie
Universitätsklinikum Charité, Berlin

Professor David Cella, PhD
Northwestern University
Center on Outcomes Research and Policy Studies
Evanston, IL, USA

Professor Dr. med. Volker Diehl
Direktor der Medizinischen Klinik I
Universität zu Köln

PD Dr. med. Andreas Dietz
Universitäts-HNO-Klinik
Heidelberg

Dr. med. Fernando Dimeo
Institut für Sportmedizin
Freie Universität Berlin

Dr. med. Wilfried Eberhardt
Innere Klinik und Poliklinik
Universitätsklinikum Essen

Dr. med. Henning Flechtner
Oberarzt der Klinik für Psychiatrie und
Psychotherapie des Kindes- und Jugendalters
Universität zu Köln

Prof. Dr. med. Manfred Heim
Chefarzt Sonnenbergklinik
Bad Sooden-Allendorf

Michel Henry-Amar, MD
Registre Général des Tumeurs du Calvados &
Service de Recherche Clinique
Centre François Baclesse
Caen, France

Dr. med. Bernhard Holzner
Psychiatrische Abteilung
Universitätsklinik Innsbruck, Austria

Dr. med. Andreas Josting
Medizinische Klinik I
Universität zu Köln

Professor Stein Kaasa, MD, PhD
Chair in Palliative Medicine
Palliative Medicine Unit
Trondheim University Hospital, Norway

Heidi Knobel, PhD
Palliative Medicine Unit
Trondheim University Hospital, Norway

Timothy J. Littlewood, MD
John Radcliffe Hospital
Oxford, United Kingdom

Jon Hårvard Loge, PhD
Department of Behavioural Sciences in Medicine
University of Oslo, Norway

Line M. Oldervoll, PhD
Department of Physical Medicine and
Rehabilitation – Unit for Applied Clinical Research
Norwegian University of Science and Technology
Trondheim, Norway

Dipl.-Psych. Katrin Reuter
Abteilung für Psychiatrie und Psychotherapie
Universitätsklinik Freiburg

Dr. med. Jens-Ulrich Rüffer
Medizinische Klinik I
Universität zu Köln

Professor Dr. med. Reinhold Schwarz
Leiter der Abt. für Sozialmedizin
Institut für Arbeits- und Sozialmedizin
Universität Leipzig

Prof. Dr. med. Peter Vaupel
Institut für Physiologie und Pathophysiologie
Johannes Gutenberg-Universität Mainz

Mechteld R. M. Visser, PhD
Department of Medical Psychology
Academic Hospital University Amsterdam
The Netherlands

PD Dr. phil. Joachim Weis
Leiter der Psychosozialen Abteilung
Klinik für Tumorbiologie an der
Albert-Ludwigs-Universität Freiburg

KARGER
Fax +49 761 4 52 07 14
E-mail Information@Karger.de
www.karger.com

Artikel (Volltext) und Inhaltsverzeichnisse sowie
das vorläufige Inhaltsverzeichnis des nächsten Heftes:
www.karger.com/journals/onk/onk_bk.htm

ONKOLOGIE

Vol. 24, Suppl 2, Februar 2001

Grußwort

Sehr geehrte Gäste,

wir freuen uns sehr, Sie hier in Köln nun schon zum 2. Internationalen Symposium «Fatigue und Krebs» begrüßen zu können.

Im ersten Treffen 1999 ist es uns gelungen, eine erste Standortbestimmung vorzunehmen und die Bedeutung von Fatigue in der Tumorbehandlung transparent zu machen. Wir wissen heute, dass nahezu alle Patienten an einer der möglichen Ausprägungen von Fatigue über eine kurze oder längere Zeit leiden. Selbst Jahre nach erfolgreicher Beendigung einer Therapie sind viele Patienten durch eine deutlich erhöhte Erschöpfung beeinträchtigt. Unsere Bemühungen haben dazu beigetragen, dass Fatigue heute als Problemfeld wahrgenommen wird und eine ernsthafte Diskussion über Ursachen, Diagnose, Differentialdiagnose und Behandlung von Fatigue bundesweit stattfindet.

Gerade diese Diskussion und die neuen Entwicklungen im Bereich Fatigue haben uns motiviert, ein zweites Symposium zu veranstalten. Ziel ist es, die Erfassung von Fatigue zu vereinfachen und auch international unter einheitlicheren Gesichtspunkten zu organisieren. Die Abgrenzung und Überschneidung zu anderen Krankheitsbildern soll deutlicher werden. Insbesondere werden wir auch über den rationalen Einsatz von Erythropoetin diskutieren, um frühzeitig einen verantwortungsvollen Umgang mit dieser neuen Möglichkeit der Behandlung zu initiieren.

Um diese Ziele zu erreichen, werden wir in Zukunft Fatigue auch als Zielkriterium («therapy endpoint») von Therapie- oder Interventionsstudien mit aufzunehmen haben. Über das Wie werden wir auf diesem Symposium einiges erfahren können.

Wir hoffen auf eine erfolgreiche Fortsetzung der ersten Tagung, eine spannende Diskussion und im Ergebnis auf erste praktische Behandlungsansätze.

Ihre
V. Diehl H. Flechtner J.-U. Rüffer

KARGER

Fax +49 761 4 52 07 14
E-mail Information@Karger.de
www.karger.com

Accessible online at:
www.karger.com/journals/onk

Fatigue and BMT: Current Status and Future Directions

M.A. Andrykowski

Department of Behavioral Science, University of Kentucky College of Medicine, Lexington, KY, USA

Fatigue is a serious problem evidenced by survivors of blood and marrow transplantation (BMT). The majority of BMT survivors report fatigue when current physical symptoms are assessed. While typically mild to moderate in severity, fatigue can become a chronic problem and ultimately have a profound impact upon BMT survivors' quality of life (QOL). The fact that many BMT survivors do not anticipate the extent and chronicity of fatigue that they ultimately experience can further contribute to the aversiveness of the problem. Despite the prevalence, severity, and impact of fatigue, little in-depth information is available regarding the experience of fatigue in the BMT setting. The empirical research regarding the experience of fatigue in BMT survivors will be summarized. Data relevant to the prevalence, severity, correlates, chronicity, and comorbidity associated with fatigue in BMT survivors will be presented. In particular, relevant data from two multicenter studies of QOL in BMT survivors will be presented. The samples in both studies consisted of disease-free adult survivors of autologous or allogeneic BMT. All study participants were treated with BMT for a malignant disease. In the first study, BMT survivors (n = 200; minimum of 12 months post-BMT) from five BMT centers in the United States completed an initial assessment of a telephone interview and completion of a packet of questionnaires. A follow-up assessment consisting of completion of a questionnaire packet was conducted 18 months following completion of the initial assessment. Results from the questionnaire data indicated 'feeling tired' was the most prevalent (78%) and most severe (mean = 3.7 on 7-point Likert scale) physical symptom reported by BMT survivors. Results from the interview data indicated that current problems with 'energy level' were reported by 65% of BMT survivors. The majority of problems (70%) with energy level were 'mild' in severity while an additional 20% were rated as 'moderate' and the remaining 10% were rated as 'severe'. The extent of current problems with energy level was highly related to ratings of current functional QOL with more severe energy level problems associated with poorer QOL. The extent of current problems with energy level was not associated with current reports of anxious or depressed mood. Analysis of both questionnaire and interview data indicated that reports of current fatigue and energy level were not significantly associated with demographic (age, gender, education) or clinical variables (TBI, disease stage at BMT, type of BMT, time post-BMT, diagnosis). Finally, results of both cross-sectional and longitudinal analyses indicated that problems with fatigue and energy level did not generally abate with the passage of time. In a second study of BMT survivors (n = 110; minimum of 2 months post-BMT), all participants completed a telephone interview. All respondents were ambulatory and living at home. The majority (57%) reported that 'energy level' was a significant current concern while an additional 34% reported that 'energy level' was no longer a significant concern but had been a concern at some time following BMT. Significantly, energy level concerns did not appear to decrease with time. No significant differences in the prevalence of energy level concerns was evident among BMT survivors < 12 months post-BMT, 12–24 months post-BMT, and 24–72 months post-BMT. Mean current energy level was described as approximately 68% of individuals pre-BMT energy level with current energy level described as 'much less' than pre-BMT levels by about 40% of BMT survivors. It is concluded that while fatigue is clearly a problem in BMT survivors, further research is clearly warranted. Future research must avoid the methodological problems characteristic of much of the research with BMT survivors to this point in time: small sample sizes, lack of appropriate comparison groups, and reliance on single-item or poorly developed measures of fatigue. In particular, researchers are encouraged to explore the utility of including biological or physical indices that could reflect upon the problem in fatigue in BMT survivors. Substantively, future research should move away from simple documentation of the prevalence and severity of fatigue and focus upon the biological and psychosocial factors responsible for the occurrence and maintenance of fatigue. The ultimate goal of research in this area should be the development of biological or behavioral interventions with demonstrable success in preventing or managing the experience of fatigue in BMT survivors.

The Results of a Systematic Review of r-HuEPO on Fatigue in Cancer Patients

A. Bottomley

EORTC Data Center, Bruxelles, Belgium

Fatigue is an increasing problem facing cancer patients and a problem gaining worldwide attention both among patient groups and the health care community. Over the last decade, an increasing number of studies support the use of recombinant human erythropoietin (r-HuEPO). This treatment can be effective in alleviating anemia in patients with inadequate levels of endogenous r-HuEPO. In non-oncology studies, a number of papers suggest r-HuEPO not only reduces anemia, but also improves fatigue and patient QL. Generally, oncological research suggests that r-HuEPO can, in some respondents, lead to a reduction of anemia. However, it is not known for certain whether r-HuEPO benefits such as reduced fatigue and improved QL, occurring in non-cancer patients, are evident in oncology patients. Given cancer patients experience significantly different pathological, clinical and psychosocial concerns, many of the results relating to r-HuEPO-induced fatigue levels and QL improvements in non-cancer patients cannot be assumed for oncology patients. For example, anemia is common in cancer patients, particularly when undergoing treatment with cytotoxic agents, and is frequently witnessed accompanying paclitaxel, single treatments with carboplatin, as well as combined paclitaxel-carboplatin treatments. Because anemia can be a side effect of radiotherapy, the complexities of cancer patient treatment and psychological adjustments cannot be compared to those of other diseases. Further, cancer patients suffering from anemia experience fatigue, along with other problems: shortness of breath, headaches, impaired mobility, dizziness, chest pain, loss of sexual desire, and reduced motivation. Therefore, the effect of r-HuEPO on cancer patients' fatigue and QL is relatively unknown.

The method of review required two reviewers to independently identify all studies. Study identification was based on searches of various databases including hand journal searchers. Minimum requirements were set for the studies to be eligible for inclusion in the review, and both RCT and non-RCT were included. To evaluate the methodological quality of selected articles, a coding scheme was developed. A total of 13 studies are critically reviewed.

The results of the review suggest that there were methodological problems with many of the studies identified. Problems were evident in all aspects of design, from selection of appropriate tools to statistical analysis, presentation, and clinical interpretation of results. These issues will be fully detailed during the presentation.

In conclusion, it is argued that the weaknesses in the designs of past studies make it difficult to draw robust conclusions about the effect of r-HuEPO on fatigue and QL. Clinicians increasingly use r-HuEPO, not only to improve levels of hemoglobin and reduce transfusion requirements, but also to reduce symptoms such as fatigue and to improve QL. However, it is believed that while there is some evidence for gains in improved fatigue and QL for some patients using r-HuEPO, in general this has not been adequately documented, and more reliable research is urgently needed to validate the effects of r-HuEPO on fatigue and QL.

Einfluss des Hämoglobinwertes auf die Prognose von Patienten mit lokal fortgeschrittenen Kopf-Hals-Tumoren – Ergebnisse einer deutschen randomisierten Multicenterstudie

V. Budach

Universitätsklinikum Charité, Campus Charité Mitte, Klinik für Strahlentherapie, Berlin, Germany

Ziele: Niedrige Hämoglobinwerte werden in verschiedenen klinischen Studien immer mit ungünstigen Therapieergebnissen in Verbindung gebracht. Im Rahmen einer großen deutschen Multicenterstudie, in die Patienten aus 10 deutschen Kliniken eingebracht wurden, untersuchten wir den Einfluss des Hb-Wertes auf die lokale Tumorkontrolle, das progressions- und metastasenfreie sowie das Gesamtüberleben.

Material und Methoden: Die Behandlung in den beiden Studienarmen bestand aus einer hyperfraktionierten, akzelerierten Radiotherapie mit einer Gesamtdosis von 77,6 Gy (Arm A) bzw. 70,6 Gy (Arm B). Die Fraktionierung im Studienarm A betrug 14 Gy mit täglichen Einzeldosen von 2 Gy, anschließend wurden 63,6 Gy mit 2× 1,4 Gy bis zu einer Gesamtdosis von 77,6 Gy appliziert. Im Studienarm B wurden während der ersten 3 Wochen 30 Gy mit 2 Gy täglich und anschließend 40,6 Gy mit 2× täglich 1,4 Gy (Gesamtdosis: 70,6 Gy) eingesetzt. Bei beiden Verfahren wurde eine Gesamtbehandlungszeit von 40 Tagen eingehalten, um den Einfluss unterschiedlicher Repopulierungsraten der Tumorstammzellen zu minimieren. Im Studienarm B wurde zusätzlich Mitomycin C (10 mg/m^2) an den Tagen 5 und 36 sowie 600 mg/m^2 5-FU an den Tagen 1–5 (120 Std. c.i.) gegeben. Das Zielvolumenkonzept beinhaltete bei makroskopischen Tumoren bzw. Lymphknoten 77,6 Gy (A) bzw. 70,6 Gy (B). Im Zielvolumen 2. und 3. Ordnung wurden 60 Gy/50 Gy unabhängig vom Behandlungsarm appliziert.

Ergebnisse: Der mittlere Nachbeobachtungszeitraum für insgesamt 384 Patienten betrug 30 Monate. Das Durchschnittsalter war 54,5 Jahre, die Geschlechtsverteilung war 82% Männer gegenüber 18% Frauen. Die Tumorlokalisation verteilte sich prozentual auf 60,4%

Oropharynx (n = 232 Patienten), 32,2% Hypopharynx (n = 124) und 7,3% Mundhöhle (n = 28). Nach der TNM-Klassifizierung waren zum Zeitpunkt der Diagnosestellung 94,5% (n = 363) aller Fälle Tumoren im Stadium IV und nur 5,5% (n = 21) im Stadium III, was die lokal weit fortgeschrittenen Tumorstadien bei diesen Patienten unterstreicht. Stratifikationskriterien für die Studie waren Tumorlokalisation, Lymphknotenstatus und die teilnehmenden Kliniken.

Die hier dargestellten Ergebnisse wurden nach dem «Intent-to-treat»-Prinzip ermittelt. Unter Schätzung der Überlebenszeiten nach Kaplan und Meier betrug die lokoregionäre Tumorkontrolle nach 2 Jahren 46,4% (A) bzw. 57% (B) (HR: 0,72, 95% CI: 0,53–0,98), die Gesamtüberlebenszeit 39,1% (A) bzw. 49,4% (B) (HR: 0,80, 95% CI: 0,62–1,04). Die Raten für Metastasenfreiheit (Arm A: 63,0% vs. Arm B: 64,6%) und progressionsfreies Überleben (Arm A: 33,7% vs. Arm B: 40,0%) waren in den beiden Behandlungsarmen statistisch nicht signifikant unterschiedlich.

Im Hinblick auf akute Nebenwirkungen und Spätfolgen der Radiatio konnten in beiden Behandlungsarmen keine Unterschiede beobachtet werden, so dass beide Therapieverfahren als isoeffektiv angesehen werden können.

Ein Hb-Wert ≤14 g/dl erwies sich in der univariaten Analyse mit dem Log-Rank-Test als unabhängiger prognostischer Faktor für die lokoregionäre Tumorkontrolle (p = 0,003; Arm A: 35,0% vs. Arm B: 56,8% nach 2 Jahren) und das Gesamtüberleben (p = 0,036; Arm A: 28,4% vs. Arm B: 45,3% nach 2 Jahren). Der Hb-Wert hatte keinen Einfluss auf die Metastasenfreiheit und das progressionsfreie Überleben. Bei Hb-Werten >14 g/dl wurde zwischen beiden Behandlungsarmen kein Unterschied beobachtet. Im Studienarm A bestand ein statistisch hochsignifikanter Unterschied zwischen den Hb-Werten >14 g/dl vs. ≤14 g/dl bezüglich der lokoregionären Tumorkontrolle (p = 0,002; Hb ≤14 g/dl: 35,0% vs. >14 g/dl: 57,4% nach 2 Jahren), progressionsfreiem Überleben (p = 0,010; Hb ≤14 g/dl: 26,6% vs. >14 g/dl: 40,4% nach 2 Jahren) und Gesamtüberleben (p = 0,001; Hb ≤14 g/dl: 28,4% vs. >14 g/dl: 49,4% nach 2 Jahren). Im Behandlungsarm B waren derartige Unterschiede nicht nachzuweisen. Auch nach multivariater Adjustierung der Ergebnisse nach Geschlecht, TNM-Stadium, histologischem Grading und Tumorsitz mit dem proportionalen Hazard-Modell von Cox waren die adjustierten p-Werte mit p = 0,002, p = 0,01 bzw. p = 0,001 stabil. Die korrespondierenden Hazard-Raten lagen bei 0,51 (0,30–0,88), 0,57 (0,35–0,93) bzw. 0,55 (0,34–0,89).

Folgerung: Nach diesen Ergebnissen erweist sich der Hb-Wert bei einem Schwellenwert von 14 g/dl als unabhängiger prognostischer Faktor für die lokoregionäre Tumorkontrolle, das progressionsfreie und das Gesamtüberleben. Der o.g. Hb-Wert bestätigt sich als unabhängiger Prognosefaktor für die alleinige akzeleriert hyperfraktionierte Bestrahlung (Arm A), nicht jedoch für die Radiochemotherapie (Arm B). Eine mögliche Schlussfolgerung könnte sein, dass durch Mitomycin C der prognostische Einfluß von Hb-Werten <14 g/dl ausgeglichen werden kann.

Autoren: V. Budach[1], S. Dinges[2], K. Haake[2], M. Stuschke[3], H. Sack[3], K.-D. Jahnke[4], M. Baumann[5], T. Herrmann[5], W. Budach[6], M. Bamberg[6], R. Sauer[7], R. Felix[8], W. Hinkelbein[9], H. Frommhold[10], J. Dunst[11], M.-L. Sauter-Bihl[12], K.-D. Wernecke[13]

Strahlenkliniken Campus [1]Mitte und [8]Wedding, [2]HNO-Klinik, UK Charité, Berlin; [3]Strahlenklinik und [4]HNO-Klinik, UK Essen; Strahlenkliniken: [5]UK Dresden, [6]UK Tübingen, [7]UK Erlangen, [9]UK Benjamin-Franklin, Berlin; [10]UK Freiburg, [11]UK Halle, [12]GH-Karlsruhe, [13]Institute for Medical Biometry, Berlin, Germany

Fatigue Assessment in Multi-Lingual Clinical Studies

D. Cella

Evanston Northwestern Healthcare and Northwestern University, Evanston, USA

Fatigue is common among cancer patients. There are now several options available for assessing fatigue in cancer patients. These options include linear analog assessment and the Functional Assessment of Cancer Therapy (FACT) Fatigue Scale, which comprises 13 of 20 questions used to assess patient concerns associated with cancer-related anemia. Several clinical trials have demonstrated that treatment of anemia may lead to improvement not only in levels of fatigue, but in more general measures of quality of life (QOL) as well. The effect of Epoetin alfa on QOL has been assessed in a number of trials. In the largest randomized trial, Epoetin alfa-treated patients experienced significant improvements in fatigue and cancer-specific QOL as measured by the FACT-G. In non-randomized large community-based trials, Epoetin alfa-treated patients also experienced significant improvements in fatigue and QOL. Increase in hemoglobin was correlated with improved QOL in all trials. Clinical trials including QOL endpoints are increasingly conducted in many cultures and languages. Pooling of data across countries and cultures within such trials requires examination of language-dependent variations in QOL responses and the effect of pooling on the results of trials. QOL data from a multinational, randomized, placebo-controlled clinical trial to assess the effect of Epoetin alfa on cancer-related anemia were analyzed to evaluate the measurement characteristics of six language versions of the Functional Assessment of Cancer Therapy-Anemia (FACT-An): Dutch, French, German, Italian, Portuguese, and English. Classical test theory and item response theory were used to test for internal consistency and differential item functioning (DIF), respectively, across the different language versions. Traditional measures of reliability showed that internal consistency was high across all languages for both of the clinical trial's FACT-An derived primary endpoints: FACT-G total (range: 0.83–0.91) and the Fatigue subscale (range: 0.89–0.92). Using English as the reference language, Rasch rating scale analysis was used to perform pairwise comparisons for each of the five target languages. The analysis generated relative item location hierarchies for each language with a criterion of >0.5 logit used to define DIF. Results revealed 21 of 200 (10.5%) cases of DIF for the FACT-G and Fatigue items. An 89.5% item location invariance justified pooling of data for the primary endpoint analyses. All-item endpoint analysis can then be compared to 'invariant-item-only' endpoint analysis to support the decision. Future challenges include defining conditions (e.g., degree of DIF) under which language or culture variation may be too excessive to support pooling, and how to interpret multicultural trial results when the same questions perform differently across languages or cultures.

Tumor Oxygenation and Hb

A. Dietz

Universitäts-HNO-Klinik Heidelberg, Germany

Introduction: The pre-therapeutic hemoglobin level (Hb) has been postulated to constitute a prognostic marker for outcome after primary chemoradiation of patients with advanced cancer of the head and neck. However, this hypothesis has not been tested systematically in large study samples.

Patients and Methods: In the years of 1992 to 1997, 125 patients with advanced head and neck cancer (st. III/IV UICC) were treated with primary chemoradiation in two different prospective multicentric trials, 62 patients in trial A (phase II, 1992–1995), and 63 patients in trial B (phase III, 1995–1997). Beside initial Hb, other pre-therapeutic parameters with potential prognostic relevance were assessed and correlated with clinical outcome after 43 months follow-up: total tumor volume (TTV; calculated in initial CT-scans), tumor oxygenation (polarographic measurements with Eppendorf-Histography), TNM, tumor localisation, age and performance status.

Results: The evaluation of the clinical endpoints progression-free and overall survival and local tumor control, revealed that Hb and TTV were independent parameters with strong predictive character for outcome after primary chemoradiation in both trials (n = 125). Bivariate analysis showed for Hb < Median [13.5g/dl] a Hazard-Ratio of 2.1 [p = 0.002]; and for TTV > Median [98 ml] a Hazard-Ratio of 2.0 [p = 0.006]. Severe anemia (Hb < 10g/dl) was an adverse factor in 3 patients. Hypoxia was associated with poorer initial therapeutical response but was not predictive for clinical outcome. Furthermore, tumor oxygenation showed no correlation with Hb. The other parameters examined failed to show prognostic significance.

Conclusion: Our results indicate a high prognostic value of initial Hb for outcome after primary chemoradiation in advanced head and neck cancer and imply a therapeutic benefit of Hb-substitution or erythropoietin administration. We propose to test this in randomized clinical trials.

Exercise as Therapy for Cancer Fatigue: When Should Rehabilitation Start?

F. Dimeo

Institute of Sports Medicine, Freie Universität Berlin, Germany

Fatigue is a frequent and serious problem of patients with oncological and haematological diseases. Several studies have shown that this symptom may affect more than 60% of the patients during therapy. Furthermore, fatigue may be a long-lasting problem and persist for months, even years, after concluding treatment. This symptom may be related to the loss of physical performance experienced by cancer patients. In fact, cancer and its treatment frequently generate several anatomical and functional changes (anaemia, reduction of vital capacity, impairment of left ventricular function, loss of muscle mass and of plasma volume, increased production of inflammation mediators) which may result in a severe loss of physical performance. Due to the loss of physical performance, light physical efforts results in these patients in dyspnea, tachycardia and muscle soreness. To reduce discomfort, patients are then advised to avoid physical effort and to reduce the level of physical activity. However, the result of these empirical measures can be paradoxical. Cancer patients reduce physical efforts to a minimum and avoid activities like stair climbing or walking for prolonged periods. This lack of physical activity generates a severe loss of muscle mass and a further impairment of cardiorespiratory function. Therefore, a self-perpetuating condition of easy tiredness, reduced activity and further impairment of physical performance is created. We have previously reported that aerobic exercise is an effective method to reduce fatigue and to increase performance status in cancer patients. Physical activity generates an increase of muscle mass and an improvement in cardiovascular work capacity; therefore, less effort is necessary to manage everyday activities. Nevertheless, the effects of exercise are not limited to an improved performance status or to a higher quality of life: aerobic training has been shown to reduce the severity of secondary effects and to accelerate bone marrow regeneration in patients undergoing high-dose chemotherapy with peripheral stem cell rescue.

Recent studies have shown that exercise programmes may also improve the physical performance and quality of life of cancer patients after surgery and of patients with haematological neoplastic diseases during conventional and intensive therapies. Furthermore, some evidence suggest that exercise may result in an increased production of haematopoetic growth factors.

Correction of Anemia in Patients with Locally Advanced Non-Small Cell Lung Cancer (NSCLC) Receiving Combined-Modality Treatment: First Study Results and Outlook for Future Investigations

W. Eberhardt

University of Essen Medical School, Essen, Germany

Combined modality treatment has emerged as a standard of care for selected patients subgroups of NSCLC stages IIIa and IIIb [1]. Several possibilities to combine the different therapeutic modalities chemotherapy, radiotherapy and surgery have been tested and, up to now, a clearly optimal approach has not been described. Of these, combinations including preoperative cisplatinum-based chemotherapy (CTx) together with preoperative chemoradiation followed by surgery represent the most intensified treatment protocols for locally advanced non-small cell lung cancer (NSCLC), so far. First reports of feasibility and efficacy with these combinations have been published [2] and look promising, especially long-term results [3].

In our Essen treatment program, NSCLC patients of stages IIIA(N2) and IIIB usually undergo three cycles of induction CTx, then receive a concurrent chemoradiation based on hyperfractionated accelerated radiotherapy and, if possible, are taken to thoracotomy for surgical resection of the residual tumor mass.

Modern chemotherapy protocols combining platinum with newer drugs such as vinorelbine, gemcitabin and the taxanes show in general lesser hematological toxicities on leucocytes than the formerly widely employed cisplatinum/etoposide regimen. However, profound treatment induced anemia due to the included platinum agents still remains one of the major toxicities in this setting, especially, if a sequential treatment design with upfront induction chemotherapy cycles is chosen. Recent data indicate, that anemia following the first cycles might lead to tumor/tissue hypoxygenation and thus to a reduced efficacy of radiation therapy in this setting4. Therefore, searching for ways to ameliorate anemia in these protocols is believed to increase treatment efficacy, improve treatment compliance and reduce possible cardiovascular events in these high risk patients groups [4].

These were the main reasons for us to study a prophylactic use of epoetin alpha within our Essen protocol. The treatment includes three cycles of induction chemotherapy with cisplatin and paclitaxel (cisplatin [P] [50 mg/m^2 D 1+7] and paclitaxel [T] [175 mg/m^2 D 1]), given every 3 weeks. This is followed by a block of concurrent chemoradiation (P/Etoposide [100 mg/m^2 D 3,4,5]) and thoracic radiotherapy (45 Gy in 3 weeks, 1.5 Gy bid). After restaging, including repeated mediastinoscopy, we perform surgery in any case of resectability. Supportive epoietin alpha is given at three times 10,000 IU per week from the first week until the end of chemoradiation. Dosage adjustments are made due to the achieved hemoglobin levels and the aimed target is a range between 13 and 15 g/l.

Up to now, fourteen patients with NSCLC stages IIIa and IIIb have been entered to this ongoing trial. Preliminary results indicate that a) treatment is well tolerated and b) hemoglobin levels in the majority of patients can be kept well within the planned target range. The study continues up to a patient number of 30 and is meant to look at a) achievable resectability rates and b) overall survival duration in this patient group.

References

1 Mountain CF. Revisions in the International System for Staging Lung Cancer. Chest 1997; 111(6): 1710–7.

2 Eberhardt W, Wilke H, Stamatis G, et al. Preoperative chemotherapy followed by concurrent chemoradiation therapy based on hyperfractionated accelerated radiotherapy and definitive surgery in locally advanced non-small-cell lung cancer: mature results of a phase II trial. J Clin Oncol 1998; 16(2): 622–34.
3 Albain K, Rush V, Crowley J et al. Long-term survival after concurrent cisplatin/etoposide plus chest radiotherapy followed by surgery in bulky, stages IIIA(N2) and IIIB non-small cell lung cancer: 6-year outcomes from Southwest Oncology Group study 8805. Proc Am Soc Clin Oncol 1999; 18 [Abstract 1801].
4 Lee JS, Komaki R, Touroutolou N et al. Erythropoietin prevents anemia during concurrent chemoradiation therapy for locally advanced inoperable non-small cell lung cancer. Proc Am Soc Clin Oncol 1998; 17 [Abstract 1780].

The Concept 'Fatigue'

H. Flechtner[1], J.-U. Rüffer[2]

[1] Clinic for Child and Adolescent Psychiatry,
[2] Department of Internal Medicine I, University of Cologne, Germany

As some time ago with the development of concepts regarding the topic of quality of life fatigue is a quantifiable, multidimensional concept and subdomains include at least a physical, cognitive, and mental dimension. The aspects of the physical dimension are certainly related to symptoms of the disease, side effects of treatment, and acute or chronic limitations in physical activity, self care, mobility, sleep, body image etc., and in general energy (fatigue in an explicit sense). It is to date still very unclear if the further domains like cognitive and mental aspects relate more to the broad area of depressive symptoms or if they constitute a distinct and separate entity within fatigue. Since fatigue seems to be in essence a subjective phenomenon and not dependent on physical health the conceptualisation shows some inconsistencies. In regard to mental and cognitive aspects fatigue seems very much to be something along the lines of a quality of life subdomain: a subjective perception of well-being or reduction in function in well defined domains, operationalised in a set of items with different grades of difficulty or symptomatology. The physical dimension however is more clearly related to direct treatment effects and limitations coming from e. g. radiotherapy or chemotherapy and in that sense represents – at least for times under treatment or shortly after end of therapy – a mixture of subjective and objective features. This is different from quality of life aspects which are also at certain times obviously dependent on treatment effects but due to the well known and established distinction between functional and symptom scales within the instruments patients report limitations in e. g. physical functioning which is related to treatment effects or report physical fatigue as a symptom of treatment of cancer. Within quality of life all different aspects can one way or the other be related to a notion of global quality of life and remain in that respect strictly dependent on the subjective perception of the patient. This seems not entirely the same for a concept of fatigue which is also confronted with the more objectively based features of certain domains of fatigue. Another important conceptual aspect is related to the question of interventions since the subdomains almost automatically constitute or refer to areas of possible interventions. Main aim of the contribution is trying to clarify on the basis of the available empirical data how a concise concept of fatigue in the light of the mentioned difficulties could look like and how one could conceptualise different subdomains also in regard to assessment and intervention. In particular overlaps with the known quality of life concepts and with the concepts of mental illnesses like depression will be dealt with. An attempt will be made to demonstrate how the concepts of fatigue have developed during the time since the first Cologne symposium on fatigue and cancer in September 1999.

Fatigue in der Rehabilitation von Tumorpatienten

M.E. Heim, I. Özkan, O. Krauß

Sonnenberg-Klinik Bad Sooden-Allendorf, Universität Göttingen; Institut für Sozialmedizin, Universität Leipzig, Germany

Chronische Erschöpfung und Müdigkeit (Fatigue) ist als Krankheits- und Therapiefolge ein häufiges Problem in der onkologischen Rehabilitation und beeinträchtigt Lebensqualität und die berufliche Leistungsfähigkeit. Ein Ziel der komplexen Therapiemaßnahmen in der stationären onkologischen Rehabilitation ist die Besserung der chronischen Fatigue. In einer Längsschnittstudie an 180 Brustkrebspatientinnen wurden die Effekte der stationären Rehabilitation auf die gesundheitsbezogene Lebensqualität nach 4 und 12 Wochen überprüft. Es zeigte sich eine signifikante Besserung des Global Health Score und verschiedener Funktionsskalen sowie der Symptomskala Fatigue im QLQ-C30, die auch im follow-up noch nachweisbar war.
In einer Folgestudie an 247 Patienten mit verschiedenen Tumorerkrankungen wurde neben dem EORTC-QLQ-C30 und dem HADS der Fatigue-Fragebogen MFI am Beginn und nach Abschluss der Rehabilitation einge-

setzt. Bei einem Großteil der Patienten war eine Fatigue-Symptomatik bei Therapiebeginn nachweisbar und klinisch relevant. Bis zum Ende der Rehabilitation nahmen die Werte in den MFI-Skalen Allgemeine Erschöpfung und Reduzierte Motivation signifikant und relevant ab (keine Effektgrößen). Lebensqualitätsdaten verbesserten sich signifikant in allen Funktionsskalen des QLQ-C30 und in einigen Symptomskalen. Die klinische Bedeutsamkeit dieser Rehabilitationseffekte wird diskutiert. Relevante Einflüsse auf Fatigue und Zusammenhänge zwischen Fatigue und Lebensqualität im Verlauf einer onkologischen Rehabilitation werden beschrieben.

Fatigue in Cancer Survivors

M. Henry-Amar, F. Joly

GRECAN-EA 1772 and Calvados Tumour Registry Centre François Baclesse, Caen, France

From 1995 to 1998, four consecutive population based case-control studies were conducted in the Calvados area in France. They concerned Hodgkin's disease (93 cases and 186 controls), testicular cancer (71 and 119), prostate cancer (71 and 71), and breast cancer (140 and 147) survivors [1–4]. Quality of life assessment was made using the EORTC QLQ-C30 core questionnaire. Median age at interview was 40 (range 19–85) years, 47 (range 28–67) years, 73 (range 56–88) years, and 54 (range 30–70) years in the 4 groups, respectively. In cases, the median follow-up time since diagnosis was 10 (range 5–17) years in Hodgkin's disease, 10 (range 6–20) years in testicular cancer, 4 (range 3–8) in prostate cancer, and 8 (range 4–19) years in breast cancer patients. Mean fatigue scale scores were similar in cases and in controls in all groups but Hodgkin's disease where cases expressed higher fatigue than controls ($p = 0.03$). Cases and controls were grouped according to their fatigue scale score: 0 to 19 (almost normal), 20 to 39, and ≥40 (clearly abnormal). The proportion of cases with high fatigue level (≥40) was 29% (26% in males, 32% in females) in Hodgkin's disease, 16% in testicular cancer, 14% in prostate cancer, and 20% in breast cancer while, in controls, it ranged from 16 to 18%. With logistic regression taking into account gender, age at interview, tumour type, and follow-up since diagnosis, only Hodgkin's disease predicted for high fatigue level (Odds ratio = 2.3, $p = 0.016$).

Functional scale scores as well as symptom scale scores were compared according to fatigue level after adjustment on age, follow-up time since diagnosis and gender where appropriate. Physical functioning, role functioning, and emotional functioning scale scores were significantly ($p < 0.01$) lower in cases who reported higher fatigue scale scores in all groups. Social functioning scale score was also significantly ($p < 0.01$) lower in cases with high fatigue level but not in testicular cancer survivors. Similarly, global quality of life scale score was significantly ($p < 0.001$) lower in cases with high fatigue level but not in prostate cancer survivors. Concerning symptoms, a high fatigue level correlated ($p < 0.01$) with increased dyspnea scale score in all groups. It correlated ($p < 0.01$) with pain, sleep disturbance, appetite loss, and financial difficulties in Hodgkin's disease survivors; and with nausea-vomiting, pain, and appetite loss in testicular, prostate, and breast cancer survivors.

We conclude that chronic fatigue does influence quality of life in survivors of cancer, in both sexes whatever their age. The instrument used, however, does not permit to analyse the various fatigue components since fatigue is a complex entity including social, psychological, physical and biological dimensions. A more appropriate instrument, such as the Multidimensional Fatigue Inventory [5], could help assessing fatigue in these patients.

References

1 Joly F, Henry-Amar M, Arveux P, Reman O, Tanguy A, Peny AM, Lebailly P, Macé-Lesec'h J, Vié B, Génot JY, Busson A, Troussard X, Leporrier M. Late psycho-social sequelae in Hodgkin's disease survivors: A French population-based case-control study. J Clin Oncol 1996, 14(9): 2444-2453.

2 Joly F, Brune D, Couette JE, Lesaunier F, Héron JF, Pény J, Henry-Amar M. Health-related quality of life and sequelae in patients treated with brachytherapy and external beam irradiation for localized prostate cancer. Ann Oncol 1998, 9:751-758.

3 Joly F, Héron JF, Kalusinski L, Bottet P, Brune D, Allouache N, Macé-Lesec'h J, Couëtte JE, Peny J, Henry-Amar M. Quality of life in long-term survivors of testicular cancer: a population based case-control study. J Clin Oncol (submitted for publication).

4 Joly F, Switsers O, Génot JY, Delozier T, Lévy C, Vié B, Delcambre C, Allouache D, Ollivier JM, Rivière A, M. Henry-Amar. Long term quality of life in premenopausal women with node-negative localized breast cancer: A population based case-control study. ASCO 2001 (abstract submitted).

5 Smets EMA, Garsson B, Bonke B, et al: The Multidimensional Fatigue Inventory (MFI). Psychometric qualities of an instrument to assess fatigue. J Psychom Res 30: 315-325, 1995

Fatigue in Cancer Patients – Relations between Hb Values and Subjective Assessment

B. Holzner[1], M. Kopp[1], G. Kemmler[1], R. Greil[2], A.G. Zeimet[3], M. Raderer[4], M. Hejna[4], S. Zöchbauer[4], G. Krajnik[4], H. Huber[4], B.Sperner-Unterweger[1]

[1] Dept. of Psychiatry;
[2] Dept. of Internal Medicine;
[3] Dept. of Gynaecology, Univ. Hosp. Innsbruck;
[4] Dept. of Internal Medicine, Univ. Hosp. Vienna, Austria

Background: Fatigue is as an important parameter in the quality of life (QOL) of cancer patients. Objective of the present study was to investigate relations between blood data and subjective experience of fatigue and QOL in cancer patients presently undergoing chemotherapy.
Methods: This survey includes 58 cancer patients (21 colorectal, 23 bronchial, 14 ovarian cancer) with an average age of 59.2 +/– 10.6 years. According to their diagnosis all patients received individual chemotherapy. QOL was measured with the EORTC QLQ-C30, Fatigue with the Multidimensional Fatigue Inventory (MFI). These assessments were carried out immediately before each chemotherapy cycle. At the same time blood data (hemoglobin) were collected.
Results: Except for the first chemotherapy cycle, correlations between Hb and subscales of MFI were moderately high (Hb with general fatigue: $r = -0.42$ at cycle 2, $r = -0.44$ at cycle 3). Significant correlations were also found between Hb and certain EORTC QLQ-C30 subscales (Hb with global QOL: $r = -0.50$ at cycle 2, $r = -0.42$ at cycle 3).
Conclusion: In spite of the significant correlations found, results indicate that Hb values yielded rather incomplete information about subjectively experienced fatigue and QOL in cancer patients. This stresses the importance of assessing subjective fatigue data in cancer patients.

Fatigue in Long-Term Survivors

H. Knobel

Unit for Applied Clinical Research, Faculty of Medicine, Norwegian University of Science and Technology NTNU, Trondheim, Norway

Fatigue is probably the most common, unrelieved symptom of cancer and cancer treatment. Some groups of cancer patients experience fatigue after successful curative treatment. However, few systematical studies have addressed persisting fatigue after cancer cure. The majority of the studies have reported fatigue to be a significant problem among Hodgkin's disease survivors (HDS). The level of fatigue among HDS is reported to be 2–3 times higher as compared to the general population. A comparative study between male HDS and survivors of testicular cancer reported higher levels of fatigue and energy loss among the HDS as compared to the testicular cancer patients. Persisting fatigue is also frequently reported in long-term survivors after allogenic (BMT) and autologous stem cell transplantation (ABMT). A Norwegian study, however, failed to find any differences in fatigue level between leukemia or lymphoma patients and the general Norwegian population after BMT and ABMT. Finally, two studies of post-treatment breast cancer patients concluded that fatigue was a problem for some of the survivors but the level of fatigue was not increased compared to the general population norms.
The perception and definition of fatigue, different methodology in assessment of fatigue, the observational period and small sample sizes have to be considered when interpreting the existing data. The high prevalence of fatigue in the general population necessitates further caution.
In general, fatigue seems to be a common problem in some groups of cancer survivors. The existing studies indicate that fatigue may be related to the disease more than to late effects after the treatment per se. Systematic and comparative studies of fatigue and of possible etiologic explanations are needed to better understand why some cancer survivors experience tiredness, energy loss and memory impairment after cancer cure.

The Impact of Hemoglobin Levels on Treatment Outcomes in Patients with Cancer

T.J. Littlewood

Department of Haematology, John Radcliffe Hospital, Oxford, UK

Introduction: Anemia is a well-recognized complication of cancer and cancer treatment. The frequency of anemia in patients with cancer varies according to tumor type and treatment. Over half the patients with lymphoma, lung tumors, gynecologic, or genitourinary malignancies may develop severe anemia that would require blood transfusion, and the incidence of mild to moderate anemia in patients with solid tumors is even greater [Groopman 1999, San Miguel 1995, Coiffier 1999]. In a retrospective survey of 2719 patients with solid tumors being treated with chemotherapy, 38% had an Hb level <11.0 g/dL during the course of treatment, and 33% of the patients required at least 1 blood transfusion [Barrett-Lee 2000]. Anemia will continue to be a significant problem in overall patient management as new and more cytotoxic generations of chemotherapeutic agents are employed in combination and combined-modality regimens [Groopman 1999].

Within the past decade, results of prospective and retrospective clinical trials have shown that the impact of anemia may be more far-reaching than previously acknowledged. Beyond the signs and symptoms of fatigue, breathlessness, swollen feet, chest pain, and loss of mental acuity, anemia also significantly impairs quality of life (QOL) [Glaspy 1997, Demetri 1998, Littlewood 1999]. Furthermore, anemia has been shown to have an adverse effect on patients' life expectancy. In patients with non-small cell lung cancer, Hb level (<11.0 g/dL [Albain 1991] and <12.7 g/dL [Ohlhauser 1997]) at the time of diagnosis was one of the most important adverse prognostic factors for survival.

Treatment of Anemia: Blood transfusion has been a common approach to the correction of anemia in patients with cancer. However, blood transfusions carry significant risks including nonhemolytic transfusion reactions, hemolytic transfusion reactions, iron overload, and reduced immunocompetence [Goodnough 1999]. Reduced immunocompetence is thought to be induced by foreign proteins and may account for unfavorable survival rates in transfused patients with a variety of tumors treated surgically. To compensate for the risks associated with transfusion, the transfusion 'trigger', i.e, the level that Hb must fall to before the patient receives a transfusion, is often very low [Grogan 1999, Barrett-Lee 2000]. Unfortunately, this practice leaves anemia untreated in many patients and, as discussed previously, anemia is associated with unfavorable treatment outcomes. Furthermore, a blood transfusion will result in an immediate increase in Hb level, but the level will decrease again unless transfusion is repeated or other interventions are employed.

Epoetin alfa

About a decade ago, recombinant human erythropoietin (r-HuEPO, epoetin alfa) became available for treating anemia associated with cancer and cancer treatment. The use of epoetin alfa to increase Hb levels in patients receiving chemotherapy has been shown to improve patients' sense of well-being in randomized, controlled trials [Abels 1992, Littlewood 1999, Gabrilove 1999], and large open-label, community-based studies [Glaspy 1997, Demetri 1998]. Epoetin alfa has also been shown to effectively increase Hb levels in patients receiving radiotherapy [Lavey 1993, Lavey 1998, Dusenbery 1994, Antonadou 1998] and radiotherapy/chemotherapy combined [Glaser 1998].

The Impact on Outcomes of Correcting Anemia with Epoetin alfa: In a study of the effect of epoetin alfa on the rate of recurrence in patients with pelvic malignancies who received radiotherapy, 385 patients received epoetin alfa (n = 190) with iron supplementation, or only iron (n = 195) [Antonadou 1998]. Mean Hb level for patients who received epoetin alfa plus iron was 12.9 g/dL vs 10.6 g/dL for patients who received only iron (P = 0.0001). Importantly, there was a significantly (P = 0.007) lower rate of disease recurrence in patients who received epoetin alfa (22/190; 11.6%) compared to patients who did not receive epoetin alfa (44/195; 22.6%). The investigators concluded that the data suggest that epoetin alfa is effective in decreasing the risk of recurrence in patients with pelvic malignancies receiving radiotherapy.

A large, placebo-controlled, randomized, double-blind clinical trial of epoetin alfa was conducted in 375 anemic (baseline Hb <10.5 g/dL, or >10.5 but <12.0 g/dL following an Hb decrease of >1.5 g/dL in the previous month) patients who received nonplatinum chemotherapy for nonmyeloid hematologic and solid malignancies [Littlewood 1999, Littlewood 2000]. The original objectives of this trial were to assess the effects of epoetin alfa on transfusion requirements, Hb level, QOL, and safety. Before the study was unblinded, an additional objective was included to explore a possible relationship between increased Hb and survival. Patients were randomized to receive epoetin alfa 150–300 IU/kg body weight 3 times weekly for 12–24 weeks (n = 251), or placebo (n = 124).

Compared with placebo, patients who were treated with epoetin alfa had significantly decreased transfusion requirements (P = 0.0057), increased Hb concentration (P < 0.001), and improved QOL (P < 0.05). Median survival times were 17 months for patients who received epoetin alfa, compared to 11 months for the placebo group. The Kaplan-Meier 12-month estimates showed a trend toward better overall survival favoring the epoetin alfa group (P = 0.13; log rank test). The investigators concluded that although the study was not designed or powered for survival as an endpoint, the results suggest a survival benefit with epoetin alfa. Another trial designed to confirm a survival benefit is warranted, since other uncontrolled variables may have influenced survival, e.g., tumor stage, intensity of chemotherapy, extent of bone marrow involvement, and disease progression.

An Austrian study evaluated the effectiveness of epoetin alfa in treating anemia in 60 patients with head and neck cancer who were undergoing chemotherapy (5-fluorouracil and mitomycin C) plus radiotherapy [Glaser 1998]. Resection of the oral cavity tumor and bilateral neck dissection were carried out 5 weeks following completion of the neoadjuvant treatment. The results in the group treated with epoetin alfa (n = 30) were compared with those obtained in a group of patients who received the same anticancer regimen but were not treated with epoetin alfa (n = 30). Results showed that treatment with epoetin alfa increased Hb level and reduced transfusion requirements, and also significantly improved response rate (P = 0.009), local control (P = 0.03), and 2-year overall survival (P = 0.03).

Conclusions: The majority of physicians were trained to believe that mild to moderate anemia in patients with cancer was to be expected, and that the anemia did not cause the patient any serious harm until the Hb fell to <10.0 g/dL or even <8.0 g/dL. We now know that this theory is incorrect, and study data strongly support the notion that anemia has a negative impact on patients' QOL, and that correcting the anemia will provide an objective improvement in the patients' well-being. Data from basic science on the adverse impact of tissue hypoxia on the response to radiotherapy has now been supported by the results from clinical trials showing that hypoxic tumors do not respond as well to ionizing radiation as normoxic tumors [Hockel 1999].

Additional data indicate that anemia is one factor resulting in tumor hypoxia [Kelleher 1996], and that correcting anemia improves the response and survival chances of patients with a variety of tumors to treatment with radiotherapy with or without concomitant chemotherapy [Glaser 1998].

A study has now been reported in which patients with both solid and hematologic malignancies who received treatment with epoetin alfa seemed to have a survival advantage compared to patients treated with placebo [Littlewood 2000]. If this finding is true, and it is worth reiterating that the study was neither designed nor powered to determine survival, it still remains unclear what factors might have led to the improved survival in epoetin alfa-treated patients. A primary effect of epoetin alfa seems unlikely. Treatment with epoetin alfa, by improving patients' QOL (secondary to raising Hb) might allow the patient to receive the correct treatment doses of chemotherapy in a more timely fashion than patients who remain anemic. Improving patients' QOL may result in enhanced survival by indirect effects related to an overall sense of well-being. Lastly, treatment with epoetin alfa, by increasing Hb, may decrease tumor hypoxia with a decrease in the malignant potential of the tumor and possibly increase sensitivity to the cytotoxic medication. A combination of these hypotheses is also possible. Importantly, the old (and at times current) thinking that anemia does not matter in patients with cancer is being seriously challenged.

References

Abels RI. Use of recombinant human erythropoietin in the treatment of anemia in patients who have cancer. Semin Oncol 1992;19(3 suppl 8): 29-35.

Antonadou D, Cardamekis E, Sarris V, Tzigounia N. Effect of the administration of recombinant human erythropoietin in patients with pelvic malignancies during radiotherapy. Radiother Oncol 1998;48:S122 (abstr. 483).

Barrett-Lee PJ, Bailey NP, O'Brien MER, Wager E. Large-scale UK audit of blood transfusion requirements and anaemia in patients receiving cytotoxic chemotherapy. Br J Cancer 2000;82:93-97.

Coiffier B. Anemia associated with non-platinum chemotherapy (CT) for Hodgkin's lymphoma (HL) or non-Hodgkin's lymphoma (NHL). Eur J Cancer 1999;35(suppl 4):S331 (abstr. 1331).

Demetri GD, Kris M, Wade J, Degos L, Cella D. Quality-of-life benefit in chemotherapy patients treated with epoetin alfa is independent of disease response or tumor type: results from a prospective community oncology study. Procrit Study Group. J Clin Oncol 1998;16:3412-3425.

Dusenbery KE, McGuire WA, Holt PJ, et al. Erythropoietin increases hemoglobin during radiation therapy for cervical cancer. Int J Radiat Oncol Biol Phys 1994;29:1079-1084.

Gabrilove JL, Einhorn LH, Livingston RB, Winer E, Cleeland CS. Once-weekly dosing of epoetin alfa is similar to three-times-weekly dosing in increasing hemoglobin and quality of life. Proc Am Soc Clin Oncol 1999;18:574a (abstr. 2216).

Glaser C, Millesi W, Gossweiner S, et al. r-HuErythropoietin supply increases efficacy of neoadjuvant radiochemotherapy in patients with oral squamous cell carcinoma. Proc Am Soc Clin Oncol 1998;17:397a (abstr. 1532).

Glaspy J, Bukowski R, Steinberg D, Taylor C, Tchekmedyian S, Vadhan-Raj S. Impact of therapy with epoetin alfa on clinical outcomes in patients with nonmyeloid malignancies during cancer chemotherapy in community oncology practice. Procrit Study Group. J Clin Oncol 1997;15: 1218-1234.

Goodnough LT, Brecher ME, Kanter MH, AuBuchon JP. Transfusion medicine. First of two parts—blood transfusion. N Engl J Med 1999; 340:438-447.

Grogan M, Thomas GM, Melamed I, et al. The importance of hemoglobin levels during radiotherapy for carcinoma of the cervix. Cancer 1999;86:1528-1536.

Groopman JE, Itri LM. Chemotherapy-induced anemia in adults: incidence and treatment. J Natl Cancer Inst 1999;91:1616-1634.

Höckel M, Schlenger K, Hockel S, Vaupel P. Association between tumor hypoxia and malignant progression: the clinical evidence in cancer of the uterine cervix. In Tumor Hypoxia. Eds, Vaupel P and Kelleher DK. Wissenschaftliche Verlagsgesellschaft mbh Stuttgart 1999:65-74.

Kelleher DK, Matthiensen U, Thews O, Vaupel P. Blood flow, oxygenation and bioenergetic status of tumors after erythropoietin treatment in normal and anemic rats. Cancer Res 1996;56:4728-4734.

Lavey RS. Clinical trial experience using erythropoietin during radiation therapy. Strahlenther Onkol 1998;174(suppl 4):24-30.

Lavey RS, Dempsey WH. Erythropoietin increases hemoglobin in cancer patients during radiation therapy. Int J Radiat Oncol Biol Phys 1993;27:1147-1152.

Littlewood TJ, Bajetta E, Cella D. Efficacy and quality of life outcomes of epoetin alfa in a double blind placebo controlled multicenter study of cancer patients receiving non-platinum containing chemotherapy. Proc Am Soc Clin Oncol 1999;18: (abstr. 2217).

Littlewood TJ, Rapoport B, Bajetta E, Nortier J. Possible relationship of hemoglobin levels with survival in anemic cancer patients receiving chemotherapy. Proc Am Soc Clin Oncol 2000;19: (abstr. 2381).
Ohlhauser C, Bulzebruck H, Ebert W, et al. Prognostic factors for survival in inoperable non-small cell lung cancer. Oncology 1997; 20:126-131.
San Miguel JF, García-Sanz R, González M, et al. A new staging system for multiple myeloma based on the number of S-phase plasma cells. Blood. 1995;85:448-455.

Prevalence and Characteristics of Fatigue in Hodgkin's Disease Survivors

J.H. Loge, S. Kaasa, R. Telhaug, H. Knobel, K.A. Kvistad, L. Oldervoll

Department of Behavioral Sciences in Medicine, University of Oslo; Department of Oncology and Radiotherapy, Trondheim University Hospital; Unit for Applied Clinical Research, The Norwegian University for Science and Technology, and MR Center, Medical Division, Trondheim University Hospital, Norway

Previous studies indicate that chronic fatigue is common among survivors of Hodgkin's disease. The causality of such fatigue is poorly understood, and there is limited knowledge about the subjective health status of chronic fatigued survivors of Hodgkin's disease.
The study's aims were to assess the levels of fatigue and the prevalence of chronic fatigue in Hodgkin's disease survivors (HDS) and to evaluate the subjective health status among chronic fatigued HDS.
Fifty-three HDS from one region of Norway treated 1987–1997 filled in the Fatigue Questionnaire, the SF-36, the HADS and the Impact of Event Scale. The HDS were compared to general population norms (N = 2214) and to 459 HDS treated at another Norwegian hospital.
The HDS' fatigue scores (mean (95% CI)) were: total fatigue = 16.5 (15.0–18.0), physical fatigue = 10.9 (9.8–12.0) and mental fatigue = 5.6 (5.0–6.1). Nineteen subjects (36%, 95% CI = 22–48%) had chronic fatigue. The fatigue scores and the prevalence of chronic fatigue were higher than in the normal controls ($P < 0.001$). The fatigue scores were higher than in the other cohort of HDS ($P < 0.01$). The chronic fatigued HDS had higher levels of HADS-anxiety ($P = 0.002$) and HADS-depression ($P = 0.001$) than the non-chronic fatigued HDS. The chronic fatigued HDS (both samples combined) displayed the poorest subjective health (s-scores) in the physical scales of the SF-36 (General health = –1.47, Role physical = –1.45, Physical functioning = –1.3). The chronic fatigued normal controls had poorest mental health (s-scores: General health = –1.56, Mental health = –1.54, Social functioning = –1.47). The differences in the two latter scales reached statistical significance ($P < 0.01$).
Chronic fatigue in HDS is associated with psychological distress, but subjective physical health is mostly affected as opposed to chronically fatigued normal controls.

Aerobic Exercise Training Reduces Fatigue in Chronic Fatigued Hodgkin's Disease Survivors

L.M. Oldervoll[1], H. Knobel[2], J.H. Loge[2,3], S. Kaasa[2]

[1] Department of Physical Medicine and Rehabilitation,
[2] Unit for Applied Clinical Research, The Norwegian University of Science and Technology, Trondheim;
[3] Department of Behavioral Sciences in Medicine, University of Oslo, Norway

Introduction: The prevalence of chronic fatigue among Hodgkin's disease survivors is 25–30%, compared to 11% in the general Norwegian population. To our knowledge, no published study has tested how physical exercise effects upon fatigue in HDS.
Aim: The aims of the study was to examine effects of physical exercise upon fatigue in HDS, and the feasibility of such an intervention including compliance and effects upon aerobic capacity.
Material and Methods: Sixty-two patients with Hodgkin's disease were identified as eligible from a cohort of HDS who were treated at University Hospital in Trondheim in the period 1987–1997. Fifty-three patients (86%) returned filled-in questionnaire including the Norwegian version of the Fatigue Questionnaire (FQ). The FQ measures physical fatigue (PF) (7 items) and mental fatigue (MF) (4 items). All eleven items are designated total fatigue (TF). Nineteen subjects (36%) reported chronic fatigue (= fatigue cases). They were invited to attend further testing including medical examination, physical exercise testing and spirometry. Fifteen of the chronic fatigue subjects agreed to participate and completed the tests.
All the patients were visited in their homes and received guidance in their personal training program. They were supposed to exercise 3 times a week for 20 weeks. The work intensity of the exercise session was registered on a pulse rate register watch (Polar Sport tester). In addition all the patients were instructed to write an exercise diary. On this background they received guided comments on intensity and were motivated to continue their exercise sessions. The work intensity should be 70–85%

of their maximum heart rate. Follow-up phone calls was done regularly during the exercise period. At the end of the intervention period the patients were re-tested for aerobic capacity, fatigue and other subjective health parameters.

Results: Ten of the fifteen who had completed the tests agreed to enter an exercise intervention period for 20 weeks. One of the ten patients was excluded before starting the intervention because of relapse. Nine of the ten patients completed the study. Six of the nine patients adhered to the exercise program according to the Polar sport tester. VO_{2max} (maximal aerobic capacity) was significantly improved from 33,9 ml $kg^{-1}min^{-1}$ before the training to 36,5 ml $kg^{-1}min^{-1}$ after completing the intervention. The heart rates on standard sub maximal loads on the treadmill was also significantly reduced. Seven of the 9 patients were no longer fatigue cases after completing the intervention. Total fatigue was significantly reduced in the entire material (n = 9) reduced from 21.5 to 12.1, mental fatigue was reduced from 7.5 to 4.2 and physical fatigue from 14.0 to 7.9.

Conclusion: The present study demonstrated positive effects of aerobic exercise on chronic fatigued Hodgkin's disease survivors. However, the study is a pilot study and needs replication. The intervention was well accepted, and the majority of the patients adhered to the program as demonstrated. Aerobic exercise must therefore be considered a promising and relevant intervention against chronic fatigue in HDS.

Fatigue and/or Depression?

K. Reuter , S. Raugust, M. Härter

Department of Psychiatry and Psychotherapy, University Clinic, Freiburg, Germany

Background: Constant physical and mental fatigue are serious problems in cancer diseases. At the same time fatigue represents a keysymptom in depressive disorders. Because of phenomenological similarities and yet unknown relationships of both syndromes a further differentiation of the two concepts is necessary for clinical treatment of cancer patients and for pursuing scientific questions. From a psychodiagnostic point of view the symptoms of depressive disorders overlap with the symptoms of multidimensional fatigue. The association of fatigue and depression has been analyzed in correlation studies using self-report questionnaires based for fatigue (e.g. MFI) as well as for depression (e.g. HADS) on dimensional methodological approaches [e.g. Visser and Smets, 1998]. Up to now approaches for criteria-oriented differentiation are missing [Reuter and Härter, 2000].

Objectives: Within the first German clinical epidemiological study on the prevalence of mental disorders in cancer patients [Härter et al. 2000; Härter et al. submitted], affective disorders have been assessed according to the diagnostic criteria of DSM-IV and ICD-10. The aim of the study on differential diagnostics of depression and fatigue is first, to explore the specific symptom patterns of depressive disorders in cancer patients, thereby contributing to clarify the importance of somatic (e.g. fatigue, sleep disturbances) and psychological symptoms (e.g. self-devaluation). Second, through the additional assessment of multidimensional fatigue, severity and expression of tumor-related fatigue in patients with and without depressive disorders will be determined and discriminating symptoms and features of both disorders will be analyzed.

Methods: A total of 517 patients from inpatient and outpatient care as well as rehabilitation were first examined for current psychological distress (GHQ-12, HADS) and for life quality (SF-36). Then every second patient was asked to participate in a clinical standardized interview (CIDI), that assesses systematicely the symptoms of mental disorders and enables diagnosis according to DSM-IV. In a subsample of 210 patients the tumor-related fatigue was assessed with the Fatigue Assessment Questionnaire (FAQ) [Glaus, 1998].

Results: The lifetime prevalence for affective disorders is 26%, the current (4-week) prevalence 10%. Major depression and dysthymia are the most frequent diagnosis. The symptom profiles show that besides the leading depressive symptom depressed mood (92%), sleep disturbances (79%) decreased concentration (64%) and fatigue (60%) are the most prevalent symptoms in comorbid affective disorders and subthreshold depressive syndromes. On average the patients had 25% more somatic symptoms than psychological symptoms. A discriminant analysis demonstrated that loss of interest (b = 0.63), fatigue (b = 0.62) and psychomotor retardation or agitation (b = 0.46) are the symptoms that best discriminate between depressed and non-depressed cancer patients. The overall fatigue mean score on the FAQ was 27 (scale: 0–60). The comparison of the levels of fatigue between different diagnostic groups showed that patients with an affective disorder suffered significantly more from fatigue (mean: 36) than patients without any diagnosis (mean: 22, $p < 0.01$). The results of further discriminant analysis about the discriminating symptoms between depressive disorders and the fatigue syndrome assessed by multidimensional approach will be presented.

References

Glaus A. Fatigue in Patients with cancer. Analysis and Assessment. Recent Results in Cancer Research, No 145 Heidelberg: Springer, 1998.

Härter M, Reuter K, Schretzmann B, Hasenburg A, Aschenbrenner A, Weis J. Komorbide psychische Störungen bei Krebspatienten in der stationären Akutbehandlung und medizinischen Rehabilitation. Die Rehabilitation 2000; 39:1-7.

Härter M, Reuter K, Aschenbrenner A, Schretzmann B, Marschner N, Hasenburg A, Weis J. Psychiatric disorders and associated factors in cancer: results of an interview study with patients in inpatient, rehabilitation and outpatient treatment. Eur J Cancer (submitted).

Visser MRM, Smets EMA. Fatigue, depression and quality of life in cancer patients: how are they related? Support Care Cancer 1998; 6:101-108.

Intervention bei Fatigue: Ein mögliches Modell

J.-U. Rüffer[1], H. Flechtner[2]

[1] Medizinische Klinik I und
[2] Klinik für Kinder- und Jugendpsychiatrie, Universität zu Köln, Germany

Fatigue ist eine zunehmend Beachtung findende Nebenwirkung in der Tumorbehandlung. Durch verschiedene epidemiologischen Untersuchungen ist es gelungen, heute eine relativ genaue Abschätzung über die Prävalenz von Fatigue zu geben. Abhängig vom untersuchten Patientenkollektiv kann man davon ausgehen, dass 60–90% aller Patienten in unterschiedlichen Ausmaß von Fatigue betroffen sind. Die Auswirkungen können dabei sehr unterschiedlicher Art sein. Bekannt sind sowohl körperliche als auch mentale oder emotionale Formen der Fatigue unter denen die Patienten leiden. Wesentlich ist aber auch die Unterscheidung zwischen akuter und später Fatigue. Tritt die akute Fatigue während oder in einem unmittelbaren zeitlichen Zusammenhang zur Diagnose und Therapie auf, ist eine genaue Eingrenzung der späten Fatigue noch schwierig. Bisher ist es in nur wenigen Studien gelungen, ein homogenes Patientenkollektiv einzuschließen. Die bisherigen Daten weisen darauf hin, dass verschiedene Krankheitsentitäten ein unterschiedliches Maß an Fatigue aufweisen. Das gilt vor allem für die späte Fatigue, während die akute Fatigue eher ein Problem ist, welches alle Patienten ähnlich stark beeinträchtigt.

Um das Ausmaß von Fatigue bestimmen zu können, ist die Verfügbarkeit eines zuverlässigen Instrumentes wesentlich. Verschiedene Instrumente sind bereits zur Messung der Fatigue entwickelt und validiert worden. Ob und welches Instrument am besten Fatigue und ihre bekannten Dimensionen zu welchen Zeitpunkten erfassen kann, muss noch abschließend geklärt werden. Um in Zukunft Interventionen durchzuführen und diese wenn möglich vergleichbar zu machen, ist es allerdings wünschenswert, die am besten geeignete Erfassungsmethode zu definieren und in den entsprechenden Interventionsstudien einzusetzen.

Für mögliche Interventionsstudien gilt es zunächst diese Voraussetzungen zu berücksichtigen, um eine optimale prospektive Erfassung von Fatigue zu ermöglichen und die Effekte der eingesetzten Interventionsstrategien erheben und beurteilen zu können. Mögliche Interventionsstrategien liegen sowohl im physischen als auch im mentalen Bereich.

In diesem Beitrag wird versucht, die grundsätzlichen Voraussetzungen für eine Interventionsstudie zu beschreiben und ein mögliches Modell für solche prospektiven Studien zu entwerfen.

Fatigue in verschiedenen Bevölkerungsgruppen

R. Schwarz, O. Krauss, A. Hinz

Abteilung Sozialmedizin, Universität Leipzig, Germany

Fatigue kann Krankheitsvorläufer, Krankheitssymptom oder Ergebnis medizinischer Eingriffe sein und kennzeichnet ein besonderes Ausmaß bzw. eine spezifische Qualität von Müdigkeit und Erschöpfung. Fatigue ist ein häufiges Symptom bei vielen physischen, insbesondere chronischen Krankheiten und bei Depression, außerdem ist es Leitsymptom des Allgemeinen Erschöpfungssyndroms (General Fatigue Syndrome). Mehrwöchige Erschöpfungsphasen sind eine häufige Neben- und Nachwirkung chirurgischer, chemo- und radiotherapeutischer Behandlungen; Medikamente wie Analgetika, Psychopharmaka und Schlafmittel können tagsüber Fatigue hervorrufen. Durch Fatigue wird neben der Selbstversorgung auch die Lebensqualität von betroffenen Patienten beeinträchtigt.

Wegen der begrifflichen Nähe zwischen alltäglicher Erschöpfung / Müdigkeit und Fatigue wurde zum einen eine repräsentative Stichprobe aus der deutschen Bevölkerung (N=2037) und zum anderen eine gemischte Stichprobe aus Patienten zweier Allgemeinarztpraxen mit dem dort üblichen Krankheitsspektrum (N=724) mit dem Multiple Fatigue Inventory (MFI) und anderen Instrumenten untersucht.

Anhand der repräsentativen Stichprobe ließen sich alters- und geschlechtsspezifische Normwerte (Prozentränge) bestimmen. Frauen geben höhere Werte an als Männer; ältere Befragte höhere als jüngere. Diesen

Normwerten werden die Werte der klinischen Stichprobe gegenübergestellt. Im globalen Vergleich zeigen sich bei rund der Hälfte der Patienten deutlich erhöhte Fatigue-Werte, jedoch keine der Normstichprobe vergleichbare Alters- und Geschlechtsspezifik. Zusammenhänge zu Krankheitsmerkmalen und psychosozialen Beeinträchtigungen (ermittelt u.a. mit HADS, EORTC QLQ-C30 und Body-Mass-Index) werden beschrieben. Daran anschließend werden Überlegungen zur Bildung von Schwellenwerten (cutoff) diskutiert.

Tumor Hypoxia: Known Facts, New Insights and the Influence of Anemia

P. Vaupel[1], M. Höckel[2]

[1] Institute of Physiology and Pathophysiology, University of Mainz;
[2] Department of Obstetrics and Gynecology, University of Leipzig, Germany

Clinical investigations over the last decade on locally advanced cancer of the uterine cervix revealed median pO_2 values significantly lower than those found in the normal cervix. Tumor oxygenation was independent of patient demographics and of pretreatment tumor characteristics such as clinical size or FIGO stage and grade of differentiation. Approximately 60% of the tumors investigated contained hypoxic areas with pO_2 values $\leq$2.5 mmHg. Poor tumor oxygenation proved to be of prognostic significance for overall and disease-free survival and was associated with malignant progression [1–3]. More recent evaluations of the oxygenation status of primary and recurrent cancers of the uterine cervix have put special emphasis on the role of histology (squamous cell carcinomas, SCC vs. adenocarcinomas, AC).

pO_2 measured in primary tumors exhibited comparable oxygenation patterns for both histologies: median pO_2 = 10 mmHg, mean pO_2 = 16 mmHg, fraction of pO_2 values $\leq$5 mmHg = 36% (SCC) and 34% (AC), respectively. There were only slight differences in the fraction of pO_2 values $\leq$2.5 mmHg (23% in SCC vs. 16% in AC) and in the percentage of patients with tumor pO_2 values $\leq$2.5 mmHg (60% in SCC vs. 66% in AC). In locally recurrent tumors, no significant differences in the oxygenation status of SCC and AC were observed. For both histologies the median pO_2 was lower (SCC = 5 mmHg, AC = 6 mmHg), and the hypoxic fraction pO_2 $\leq$2.5 mmHg was higher (SCC = 37%; AC = 31%) in recurrent tumors than in primary lesions. The percentage of patients with pO_2 values $\leq$2.5 mmHg in recurrent tumors was 77% (SCC, n = 49) and 87% (AC, n = 14), respectively. Significantly better stage-for-stage prognosis for SCC than for AC of the uterine cervix thus cannot be explained by substantially different oxygenation status of the two histologies. Therefore, treatment outcome (radiation ± surgery) may additionally be influenced by parameters other than oxygenation.

In another more recent study, emphasis was put on the question of whether the pathological tumor stage (pT), rather than the FIGO stage, may have an impact on the oxygenation status. Therefore, in a subgroup of 65 patients treated with primary surgery (with curative intent), pathological tumor staging was performed based on histopathological investigation of the surgical specimens following radical hysterectomy or exenteration and lymph node dissection. This procedure identified a median maximum (histological) tumor diameter of 40 mm. In tumors with a maximum extension <40 mm (n = 37), the median pO_2 was 11 mmHg which was significantly higher than the respective pO_2 value in tumors with a maximum diameter >40 mm (n = 28, median pO_2 = 5 mmHg; $p < 0.05$). Median pO_2 values in stage pT1b tumors were significantly higher (18 mmHg) than in pT2b lesions (5 mmHg, $p < 0.05$). Hypoxic fractions were slightly lower in pT1b (bulky) tumors than in pT2b malignancies. From these data it is concluded that only a detailed histopathological tumor staging using surgical specimens enables detection of stage- and size-related differences in the oxygenation status of primary cancers of the uterine cervix. Clinical tumor dimensions and FIGO staging are not accurate enough for the estimation and characterization of the tumor oxygenation.

Besides abnormalities of the tumor microcirculation and a deterioration of the diffusion geometry, cancer-related and/or therapy-induced anemia are major causative factors for development of tumor hypoxia. Anemia and formation of carboxyhemoglobin (in heavy smokers) are a major problem in patients with tumors (tumor areas) that have a low perfusion rate. Data on the impact of anemia on the development of hypoxia are, however, somewhat controversial. In some studies, no correlation between the pretreatment hemoglobin concentration (cHb) and any of the oxygenation parameters could be found [4, 5]. However, it should be noted that only very few patients had cHb values below the normal range. In contrast, other investigations have demonstrated a (weak) association between higher hemoglobin levels and higher median pO_2 values [6, 7]. However, there are no doubts in the clinical setting that treatment of anemia (cHb <120 g/L) will provide patients with better localized tumor control and improved treatment outcome.

Traditionally, tumor hypoxia has been considered to be a therapeutic problem, as it renders solid tumors resistant to sparsely ionizing radiation, some forms of chemotherapy (e.g., cyclophosphamide, carboplatin), and photodynamic therapy. Hypoxia may also modulate the proliferation kinetics, the cell cycle position and the number of tumor cells accumulating in G0-phase through alterations of gene expression leading to proteome changes. These changes in turn can greatly modulate the amount of cells destroyed following radiation and/or chemotherapy. More recent clinical studies suggest that sustained hypoxia can additionally enhance malignant progression and may increase aggressiveness through clonal selection and genome changes. As a result, loss of differentiation and of apoptosis, chaotic angiogenesis, increased locoregional spread and enhanced metastasis can further increase resistance to therapy and can impact long-term prognosis. Multivariate analysis has shown that hypoxia is a powerful prognostic factor in cervix cancers [2,3,8], squamous cell carcinomas of the head and neck [5], and in soft tissue sarcomas [6], independent of other variables that can influence outcome.

Besides giving some indication of tumor aggressiveness, knowledge of the oxygenation status of individual tumors might be beneficial for the understanding of physiological barriers to conventional treatments and for designing specifically tailored treatment protocols for individual subjects with the aim of overcoming treatment resistance. Thus an appropriate consideration of tumor oxygenation is essential if measurement of this parameter is to be used to its full extent in terms of optimizing currently available therapeutic strategies.

References

1 Hoeckel M, Schlenger K, Knoop C, Vaupel P: Oxygenation of carcinomas of the uterine cervix: Evaluation of computerized O_2 tension measurements. Cancer Res 51: 6098-6102, 1991

2 Höckel M, Schlenger K, Aral B, Mitze M, Schäffer U, Vaupel P: Association between tumor hypoxia and malignant progression in advanced cancer of the uterine cervix. Cancer Res 56: 4509-4515, 1996

3 Höckel M, Schlenger K, Höckel S, Vaupel P: Hypoxic cervical cancers with low apoptotic index are highly aggressive. Cancer Res 59: 4525-4528, 1999

4 Rudat V, Vanselow B, Wollensack P, Bettschneider C, Osman-Ahmet S, Eble MJ, Dietz A: Repeatability and prognostic impact of the pretreatment pO_2 histography in patients with advanced head and neck cancer. Radiother Oncol 57: 31-37, 2000

5 Nordsmark M, Overgaard J: Oxygenation of Human Tumors: The Aarhus Experience. In: Vaupel P, Kelleher DK (eds) Tumor Hypoxia. Pathophysiology, Clinical Significance and Therapeutic Perspectives. pp 19-27, Stuttgart: Wissenschaftliche Verlagsgesellschaft 1999

6 Brizel DM: Human Tumor Oxygenation: The Duke University Medical Center Experience. In: Vaupel P, Kelleher DK (eds) Tumor Hypoxia. Pathophysiology, Clinical Significance and Therapeutic Perspectives. pp 29-38, Stuttgart: Wissenschaftliche Verlagsgesellschaft 1999

7 Becker A, Stadler P, Lavey RS, Hänsgen G, Kuhnt T, Lautenschläger C, Feldmann HJ, Molls M, Dunst J: Severe anemia is associated with poor tumor oxygenation in head and neck squamous cell carcinomas. Int J Radiat Oncol Biol Phys 46: 459-466, 2000

8 Hoeckel M, Knoop C, Schlenger K, Vorndran B, Baussmann E, Mitze M, Knapstein PG, Vaupel P: Intratumoral pO_2 predicts survival in advanced cancer of the uterine cervix. Radiother Oncol 26: 45-50, 1993

The Measurement of Fatigue Over Time: Response Shift in Cancer Patients

M.R.M Visser, E.M.A. Smets, M.A.G. Sprangers

Department of Medical Psychology, Academic Medical Centre, Amsterdam, The Netherlands

If patients become extremely fatigued during their treatment, they may judge the level of fatigue following this experience differently from how they would have judged it commonly. This change is referred to as response shift. Response shift is defined as a change in the meaning of one's self-evaluation of a target construct as a result of: (a) a change in the respondent's internal standards of measurement (i.e., scale recalibration); (b) a change in the respondent's values (i.e., reprioritization) (c) a redefinition of the target construct (i.e., concept redefinition)[1, 2].

For patients, response shift might be the result of adequate adaptation and might therefore be functional. For investigators, however, it poses a methodological problem concerning the measurement of change over time.

Several methods are proposed to assess the three components of response shift. These include statistical, design, individual, and qualitative approaches [2]. An example of a design approach is the 'thentest' method, which intends to measure scale-recalibration. The thentest is used in addition to the conventional pretest-posttest design. Following the completion of the posttest, patients are asked to provide a renewed judgement about their pretest levels of fatigue (thentest). Response shift is assessed by the mean difference between the pretest and the thentest scores.

Results of two studies using the thentest approach will be presented. Both studies assessed patients' level of fatigue prior to and following radiotherapy. In the first study [3], 199 patients judged their level of fatigue using a 10-point rating scale. Comparing the thentest with the pretest scores, patients retrospectively minimized their pre-treatment level of fatigue. The thentest-posttest difference was significant, whereas the conventional pretest-posttest difference was not. These results are indicative of the occurrence of response shift.

In the second study [4], 99 patients were asked to judge their level of fatigue using the Multi-Dimensional Fatigue Inventory (MFI). After the completion of the thentest, patients were interviewed about their responses. Results indicated that response shift occurred in a subsample of patients; that the thentest was valid (as indicated by its association with criterion measures of change); and that patients' verbalizations reflect response shift and mechanisms underlying response shift.
The usefulness and the validity of the thentest approach will be discussed.

References

1 Schwartz CE, Sprangers MAG (2000). Adaptation to Changing Health: Response Shift in Quality-of-life Research. American Psychological Society, Washington DC.
2 Schwartz CE, Sprangers MAG (1999). Methodological approaches for assessing response shift in longitudinal health-related quality-of-life research. Social Science and Medicine, 48, 1531-1548.
3 Visser MRM, Smets EMA, Sprangers MAG, de Haes JCJM (2000). How response shift may affect the measurement of change in fatigue. Journal of Pain and Symptom Management, 20(1), 12-18.
4 Sprangers MAG, van Dam FSAM, Broersen J, Lodder L, Wever L, Visser MRM et al. (1999). Acta Oncologica, 38, 709-718.

Neuropsychological Aspects of the Fatigue Syndrome: Conceptional Approaches and Intervention Strategies

J. Weis, M.Poppelreuter

Tumor Biology Center at the University of Freiburg, Germany

Although in the literature cancer-related fatigue is often associated with deficits in cognitive functioning and some of the multidimensional assessment instruments including a subscale of cognitive fatigue there are only a small number of papers investigating this dimension of fatigue. As a specific sequelae of the fatigue syndrome especially the domains of concentration, attention and short-term memory are affected. Although in the last decade research in psychooncology has started to focus more on the neuropsychological problems due to cancer treatment, there is still a lack of systematic studies in the field. With respect to fatigue there is an overlap between the symptoms of depression, physical exhaustion and cognitive deficits. Neuropsychological testing is required to determine and specify the prevalence rates of deficits in cognitive functioning. Especially in the rehabilitation, neuropsychological training could be an essential part of a fatigue-specific intervention program. The presentation is reviewing the problems of fatigue assessment and neuropsychological testing. First experiences with such a training program in the rehabilitation clinic of the Tumor Biology Center are reported.

ONKOLOGIE

Onkologie 2001;24:18

Hinweise für Autoren

Die Zeitschrift ONKOLOGIE ist ein Forum für alle Themen der Onkologie. Veröffentlicht werden Original- und Übersichtsarbeiten aus der internistischen Hämato-Onkologie, der chirurgischen, gynäkologischen und urologischen Onkologie, der Strahlentherapie und der klinisch-experimentellen Onkologie. Auch Beiträge zur pädiatrischen, HNO- und dermatologischen Onkologie, zu Pathologie und Biometrie, Epidemiologie, Prävention und Frühdiagnose bis hin zur psychologischen Betreuung werden berücksichtigt. Alle Beiträge unterliegen einem Begutachtungsverfahren.

1. Allgemeines, Verlagsrecht

Bitte senden Sie Ihr Manuskript in vierfacher Ausfertigung (jedes Exemplar komplett mit Abbildungen und Tabellen) direkt an den S. Karger Verlag, z. H. Dr. Heike Endemann, Postfach, D-79095 Freiburg. Eine weitere Kopie des Manuskripts soll grundsätzlich beim Autor verbleiben.

Alle Autoren müssen in einem **Begleitschreiben** durch Unterschrift bestätigen, daß die eingereichte Arbeit bislang weder ganz noch teilweise (Ausnahme: Kongreßberichte) veröffentlicht wurde noch anderweitig zur Veröffentlichung eingereicht ist und daß alle Autoren das Manuskript gelesen haben und mit der Veröffentlichung in der vorliegenden Form einverstanden sind. Es ist Sache des Autors, die Nachdruckerlaubnis für Abbildungen, Tabellen usw. aus anderen Publikationen zu beschaffen. Über die Annahme wissenschaftlicher Beiträge wird aufgrund mehrerer Gutachten entschieden (peer-review). Mit der Annahme des Manuskripts zur Publikation gehen alle Rechte auf den Verlag über. Ohne schriftliche Genehmigung des Verlages dürfen diese Publikationen oder Teile daraus nicht in andere Sprachen übersetzt oder in irgendeiner Form mit mechanischen oder elektronischen Mitteln (einschließlich Fotokopie, Tonaufnahme und Mikrofilm) reproduziert oder auf Datenträger oder einem Computersystem gespeichert werden.

Ethische und rechtliche Voraussetzungen: Zur Publikation eingereichte Manuskripte, bei denen Untersuchungen an Probanden oder Patienten durchgeführt wurden, müssen die Erklärung enthalten, daß das Versuchsprotokoll von einer Ethikkommission genehmigt wurde und den ethischen Standards der Deklaration von Helsinki in ihrer erweiterten Form von 1975 und ihren Zusätzen von 1983, 1989 und 1996 [JAMA 1997;277:925–926] entspricht. Zugleich muß im Manuskripttext auf die Einwilligung der Versuchsperson nach Aufklärung hingewiesen werden. Angaben, die auf die Identität der Person schließen lassen, sind unzulässig.

Tierversuche bedürfen gleichfalls der Genehmigung und müssen den Forderungen des Tierschutzgesetzes in seiner jeweils gültigen Fassung entsprechen. Auf diese Genehmigung ist im Manuskript hinzuweisen. Arbeiten, die nicht aus Deutschland stammen, müssen einen vergleichbaren Hinweis tragen.

Beiträge erscheinen in einer der folgenden **Rubriken:** Übersichtsarbeit, Kurze Übersicht, Originalarbeit, Laufende klinische Studie, Kurzmitteilung, Kasuistik, Brief an die Herausgeber, Kommentar, Meinung, Onkologische Fortbildung, Klinische Information, Kongreßbericht, Wilsede-Schule.

Übersichtsarbeiten, Originalarbeiten, Laufende klinische Studien, Kurzmitteilungen, Kasuistiken, Briefe an die Herausgeber, Kommentare und Editorials sind in englischer Sprache abzufassen. Alle anderen Beiträge können wahlweise in deutscher oder englischer Sprache eingereicht werden.

2. Manuskripte

Die Manuskripte sollen in $1^1/_2$zeiligem Abstand mit beidseitig je 3 cm Rand eingereicht werden. Folgender Umfang einschließlich Zusammenfassung, Abbildungen, Tabellen und Literaturzitate sollte nicht überschritten werden:

	Druckseiten	Entspricht Manuskriptseiten (einschließlich Zusammenfassung, Abbildungen, Tabellen und Literaturzitate)
Übersichtsarbeit, Originalarbeit	5	14
Kurze Übersicht, Kasuistik	3	8
Laufende klinische Studie Onkologische Fortbildung, Klinische Information	4	11
Brief an die Herausgeber	1	3
Übrige Beiträge	2	6

Für Umfangüberschreitungen wird dem Autor ein Mehrkostenanteil in Rechnung gestellt (s. unten). Kontrollieren Sie bitte das Manuskript sorgfältig auf einheitliche Bezeichnungen und korrekte Schreibweise. Typographische Gestaltung und redaktionelle Bearbeitung werden vom Verlag durchgeführt. Generelle Hinweise zur Abfassung von Manuskripten können den «Uniform Requirements for Manuscripts Submitted to Biomedical Journals» des «International Committee of Medical Journal Editors», veröffentlicht in Ann Intern Med 1997;126:36–47 bzw. http://jama.asma-assn.org/info/auinst_req.html, entnommen werden.

Manuskripte auf Diskette: Jedem Manuskript ist eine Diskette beizulegen, deren Inhalt exakt mit dem Ausdruck übereinstimmen muß. Bitte beachten Sie auch die «Hinweise für Manuskripte auf Diskette».

Bitte numerieren Sie die Seiten des Manuskripts durchlaufend, beginnend mit der Titelseite. Die Arbeit soll gegliedert sein in **Schlüsselwörter und Zusammenfassung, Key Words und Summary, Einleitung, Material und Methoden** (oder **Patienten und Methoden**), **Ergebnisse, Diskussion,** gegebenenfalls **Dank, Literatur, Tabellen, Abbildungslegenden und Abbildungen.**

Die **Titelseite** muß enthalten: **Titel und Kurztitel** der Arbeit in Deutsch und Englisch, die vollständigen Autorennamen mit der jeweiligen Institutsangabe in der Landessprache der Autoren, die vollständige Postadresse des Korrespondenzautors, gegebenenfalls mit Telefon- und Faxnummer sowie E-mail-Adresse.

Originalarbeiten müssen eine englische und deutsche **strukturierte Zusammenfassung** enthalten. Für Informationen zur Gliederung der Zusammenfassung siehe Haynes RB, Mulrow CD, Huth EJ, Altman DG, Gardner MJ: Ann Intern Med 1990;113:69–76. Die Zusammenfassungen sollen 250 Wörter nicht überschreiten und sind zu strukturieren in **Hintergrund, Material und Methoden, Ergebnisse, Schlußfolgerungen.** Die Zusammenfassung darf keine Literaturzitate, Tabellen, Abbildungen, Abbildungs- und Tabellenhinweise enthalten. Falls Hinweise auf Literaturzitate unvermeidlich sind, müssen sie vollständig sein. Zu einer Arbeit gehören 3–5 **Schlüsselwörter** (Englisch und Deutsch), die möglichst der «Medical Subjects Heading List» des Index Medicus entnommen sein sollen (die Liste ist unter www.nlm.nih.gov erhältlich). Übersichtsarbeiten folgen nicht der Gliederung von Originalarbeiten; Titelseite, Zusammenfassung, Schlüsselwörter und Literaturverzeichnis sind jedoch erforderlich.

Fußnoten sollten nur in Tabellen verwendet werden. **Abkürzungen** im Text bitte möglichst sparsam verwenden. Bei nicht allgemein üblichen Abkürzungen jeweils beim ersten Auftreten das Wort ausschreiben und die später verwendete Abkürzung in Klammern folgen lassen: z.B. Adenosin-Monophosphat (AMP). Geschützte **Produkt- bzw. Markennamen** müssen beim ersten Auftreten im Text mit einem hochgestellten ® bzw. ™ bezeichnet werden. Die Verantwortung für die korrekte Befolgung dieser Vorschrift liegt ausschließlich beim Autor. **Danksagungen** sollten unmittelbar dem Text folgen und dem Literaturverzeichnis vorangestellt sein.

Das **Literaturverzeichnis** soll nur die im Text zitierten Publikationen enthalten. Bei Übersichtsarbeiten sollten nicht mehr als 60 Literaturstellen angegeben werden, bei Kurzen Übersichten nicht mehr als 40. Die Literatur ist entsprechend der Reihenfolge des Auftretens im Text zu numerieren. Die Referenzen werden als Zahlen in eckigen Klammern in den Text eingefügt. Bitte alle Autoren einer Arbeit angeben, die Abkürzung «et al.» ist zu vermeiden. Zitiert werden sollen nur Arbeiten, die entweder publiziert oder zur Publikation angenommen sind. Der Passus «in Vorbereitung» oder «persönliche Mitteilung» ist zu vermeiden. Die Abkürzung der Zeitschriftentitel erfolgt nach dem Index-Medicus-System (www.nlm.nih.gov).

Beispiele zur Abfassung von Literaturzitaten:

(a) Zeitschriftenbeiträge: Lelie PN, Cuypers HTM, van Drimmelen AAJ, Quint WGV: Quality assessment of hepatitis C virus nucleic acid amplification methods. An international proficiency study. Infusionsther Transfusionsmed 1998;25:102–110.

(b) Bücher mit Herausgeber: Hardy WD Jr, Essex M: FeLV-induced feline acquired immune deficiency syndrome: A model for human AIDS; in Klein E (ed): Acquired Immunodeficiency Syndrome. Prog Allergy. Basel, Karger, 1986, vol 37, pp 353–376.

(c) Monographien: Schaefer UW, Beelen DW: Bone Marrow Transplantation, ed 2, revised. Basel, Karger, 1996.

In **Abbildungen** und **Tabellen** genannte Informationen bedürfen keiner Wiederholung im Text. Hinweise auf Abbildungen und Tabellen erfolgen im Text mit (Abb. 1) bzw. (Tab. 1). Abbildungslegenden sind auf einer gesonderten Seite zusammenzustellen; jede Tabelle muß eine Legende haben. Die Legenden sind kurz und präzise zu halten. **Farbabbildungen** sind möglich, erfordern jedoch einen Zuschuß des Autors zu den Druckkosten (s. unten). **Abbildungsvorlagen** sind 4fach einzureichen (Original und 3 Kopien). Auf der Rückseite der Vorlage (nicht aufkleben oder anheften) bitte den Namen des Autors, ein Titelstichwort, die Angabe, wo «oben» ist, sowie die Bildnummer angeben. Die Qualität der gedruckten Abbildungen hängt von der Qualität der Vorlagen ab.

Randomisierte, kontrollierte klinische Studien sollen nach den Empfehlungen des CONSORT-Statements [Begg C, Cho M, Eastwood S, Horton S, Moher D, Olki I, Pitkin R, Rennie D, Schulz F, Simel D, Stroup D: Improving the quality of reporting of randomized trials: The CONSORT statement. JAMA 1996;276:637–639] abgefaßt werden. Das Verfahren, nach dem die Vergleichsgruppen ermittelt wurden, muß erkennbar sein, so daß der Leser die Methode der Randomisierung nachvollziehen kann. Im Titel und in der Zusammenfassung der Arbeit ist darauf hinzuweisen, daß es sich um eine randomisierte kontrollierte klinische Studie (RCT) handelt. Wird eine RCT eingereicht, sind die «Checklist for Authors Submitting Randomized Controlled Trials» und das CONSORT-Flußdiagramm zu beachten, welche im ersten Heft jedes Jahrgangs in der englischen Version dieser Hinweise abgedruckt sind. Die CONSORT-Checklist und das CONSORT-Flußdiagramm sind auch unter www.ama-assn.org/public/journals/jama zugänglich, eine deutsche Version mit weiteren Informationen kann unter www.med.uni-muenchen.de/gmds/pub/consort.html heruntergeladen werden. Die ausgefüllte Checkliste und das Flußdiagramm müssen der Arbeit beigelegt werden, da sie in das Begutachtungsverfahren einbezogen werden.

Druckfahnen: Das lektorierte Manuskript und die Druckfahnen werden dem Korrespondenzautor zusammen mit einem Formular zur Sonderdruckbestellung zugesandt. Die Fahnen sind sorgfältig mit dem Manuskript zu vergleichen und notwendige Korrekturen auf der Fahne einzutragen. Die Korrespondenz betreffend angenommene Arbeiten und Druckfahnen bitte direkt mit dem S. Karger Verlag in Freiburg führen.

3. Kosten und Sonderdrucke

a) Sollte die Arbeit den vorgegebenen Umfang überschreiten (siehe «2. Manuskripte» und vom Autor nicht gekürzt werden, wird der Mehrumfang mit DM 650,– pro Druckseite berechnet.
b) Für Farbabbildungen wird dem Autor ein Reproduktions- und Druckkostenanteil von DM 450,– pro Abbildung in Rechnung gestellt.
c) Übersteigen die Kosten der Autorkorrektur 10% der Satzkosten, werden die Zusatzkosten dem Autor in Rechnung gestellt.

Der Korrespondenzautor erhält 25 kostenlose Sonderdrucke seiner Arbeit.

Die vollständigen Hinweise erscheinen im ersten Heft eines Jahrgangs.

KARGER

Fax +49 761 4 52 07 14
E-mail Information@Karger.de
www.karger.com

Hinweise für Autoren verfügbar unter:
www.karger.com/journals/onk/onk_gl.htm